UNVEILING THE BURDEN OF
DEAFNESS IN *INDIA*

SILENT EPIDEMIC

UNVEILING THE BURDEN OF
DEAFNESS IN *INDIA*

SILENT EPIDEMIC

Dr. Manoj Kumar Gupta

MBBS, MS (ENT)

Worldwide Published by
Pendown Press

PENDOWN PRESS LLP

An ISO 9001 & ISO 14001 Certified Co.,

Regd. Office: 3767A, Kanhaiya Nagar,
Tri Nagar, Delhi-110035
Ph.: 8130886000, 9650072927, 8595249536
E-mail: info@pendownpress.com
Branch Office: 1A/2A, 20, Hari Sadan, Ansari Road,
Daryaganj, New Delhi-110002
Ph.: 011-45794768
Website: PendownPress.com

First Edition: 2024

ISBN: 978-93-5554-951-8

Layout and Cover Designed by Pendown Graphics Team
Printed and Bound in India by Thomson Press India Ltd.

Dedication

This book is lovingly dedicated to my parents, whose unwavering support and guidance have been the bedrock of my journey. Their enduring love and encouragement have fueled my passion for making a difference in the lives of others.

In particular, I extend my deepest gratitude for the blessings they have bestowed upon me. Their belief in my abilities has been a source of strength, propelling me forward in my mission to provide compassionate care to those in need.

As I pen these words, I am acutely aware that their influence goes beyond mere dedication; it permeates every page of this book. Their wisdom, love, and invaluable support have shaped not only my personal life but also the professional path I tread, especially in the realm of healthcare.

May this book stand as a testament to the profound impact of parental love and guidance. Through their blessings, I have found the strength to illuminate the path for others, just as they have illuminated mine.

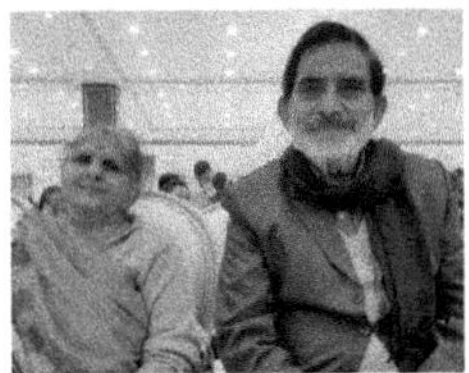

CONTENTS

ACKNOWLEDGEMENTS

In my writing journey, I extend my deepest gratitude to those whose unwavering support has been the cornerstone of both my life and the creation of this book. The realization of this endeavor is a testament to the collective encouragement, blessings, and guidance that have shaped every word on these pages.

Foremost, I express immense thanks to my life partner, Dr. Priyanka. Her unwavering belief in me has been the bedrock of my resilience through life's ebbs and flows. Her dedicated care for our home and our child has granted me the precious time to pen these thoughts. Without her, this endeavor would have been a mountain too steep to climb. Her commitment is the essence that has given Satkriti its unique character in the eyes of my patients

A debt of gratitude is owed to my mentors, particularly Sanjiv Sir and Rajeev Kapoor Sir, whose sage guidance has orchestrated transformative changes within me. Acknowledgement is also due to Akshar Yadav Sir, whose mentorship not only refined my interpersonal skills but also kindled the inspiration to embark on this literary journey.

I extend heartfelt thanks to my son, Mayank, whose steadfast love and support are the pillars on which I stand. Dr. Mouli Patel, our young, dedicated, and dynamic ENT Consultant, deserves special mention for her meticulous patient care, allowing me the freedom to craft this book.

To my dedicated team members—Ms. Manjari Mishra, Ms. Julie Gupta, Ms. Ranjana Mourya, Mr. Shishir Tiwari, and all who stood resilient during challenging times—I extend my sincere appreciation. Their unwavering dedication to our shared vision has been instrumental.

Gratitude is extended to the referring doctors, business associates, medical representatives, and pharmaceutical companies who have entrusted me and my organization with their confidence.

To my patients, your trust and faith humble me. Your unwavering belief propels me to go above and beyond in providing care.

Finally, a nod of thanks to the Universe for bestowing upon me the energy and clarity of thought needed to pen these pages. In each acknowledgment, I find a thread that weaves the tapestry of this journey—a journey enriched by the collaborative spirit of those who have touched my life.

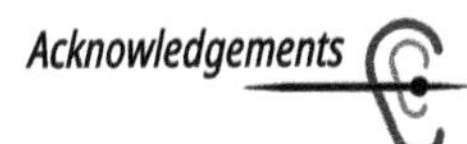

I am thankful to my friend Dinesh Verma, CEO, Pendown Press and his team for their support and suggestions throughout the creative process.

WHY THIS BOOK

I was born in the Biswanath district of Assam and completed my schooling at Sainik School Goalpara. I pursued my MS in ENT from Assam Medical College, Dibrugarh. When I was a kid, I have vivid memories of spending time with my grandfather. He used to take me to ashrams where deaf and mute people resided. Seeing their lives made me wonder: Why did God make them unable to hear and speak? As a child, I often thought about how tough it must be to live without sound and communication, and it made me feel really sorry for them. I wished that I could help them out of this misery one day.

Whenever I brought them food, they would simply nod because they couldn't hear what I was trying to communicate. My attempts to talk to them were futile, and I couldn't help but wish that someone could help them with their hearing. As I learned more about their condition, it left a lasting impression on my mind. Even as a child, giving them food and seeing their happiness brought me joy. This habit, instilled in me by my grandpa, stayed with me and molded me into a compassionate individual. I am grateful to him for teaching me the value of kindness and for shaping me into a better person.

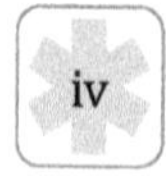

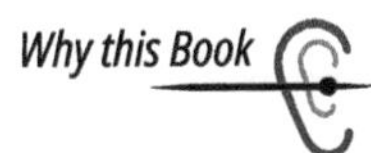

As I grew older, the tradition of offering food and gifts continued, thanks to my father, who carried on my grandfather's legacy of kindness. He used to take me to that place, but somewhere, I felt that something was missing. I used to think that food might bring moments of happiness to them, but what about the disease they were suffering from? There was a persistent feeling at the back of my mind, urging me to ask myself what more I could do to address their larger issues. This compelled me to think beyond simple gestures of goodwill.

Motivated by this big question, I chose a career in ENT medicine, focusing on Ear, Nose, and Throat health. This decision came from my inner drive to help others, especially those with hearing issues. I felt it was my duty to make a positive change. Once I entered the medical field, I did a lot of research to better understand how to assist people with hearing problems.

During my study, I found something surprising: many people didn't know that if a child is born with hearing issues and doesn't get help within the first five years, it becomes permanent, and they can't hear for the rest of their life. This discovery shook me deeply and made me even more determined to make a real difference. Now, I'm dedicated to raising awareness about early intervention for hearing problems and ensuring that no child has to live in silence if it can be prevented. Realising that the first step was to spread the word, I started a mission to inform people about this important issue, making sure we could prevent it early. At times I faced challenges and I wondered if my efforts were needed, but then I thought about my parents and grandparents, who always helped others without expecting anything in return. Their kindness and care were a part of me, pushing me to continue their legacy.

This strong desire to give back kept inspiring me in life and my medical career. I had a deep passion and motivation to do more, to create a bigger impact. I started sharing this message with everyone I met, including my patients, who, in turn, passed it onto others. However, I soon realized that this message needed to reach many, many people, and the usual ways of telling individuals about it were just too slow. That's when I did some research to find a better way to spread the word. I figured out that writing a book could help me get the message to lots of people quickly. So, I made a choice – I decided to become a writer.

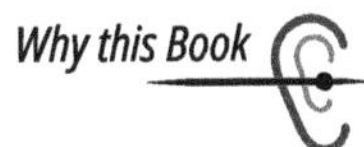

My journey as a writer started with one important goal:

"to spread awareness about this simple yet life-changing message about deafness." Even though the road ahead is tough, I pledge to stay true to my mission. Driven by the kindness in my family, writing this book is a small step towards achieving my goal to help those in need.

Case Study

Mindset Matters: How I Helped Some Friends Find Hope:

1# A new Sound for Raghav: I remember one particular day when I attended a business growth summit, where I met one of my friends, Mr. Raghav. I noticed something in his ear, so I asked him about it. He explained that he was suffering from a specific ear problem, which couldn't be cured, and it wasn't a Bluetooth device or earbuds; it was a hearing aid. I assured him that it could be treated, and that I could help him with it. In response, he was taken aback and said, "Are you joking? I've consulted many doctors in India and abroad, and they all told me it can't be cured". I then explained to him about my procedure of treatment that my first step towards treatment will be to change your mindset. I firmly believe that "if the foundation of a building is weak, the building won't stand, and it will collapse eventually. You can add more floors, but it won't work". Similarly, diseases should be treated with the right

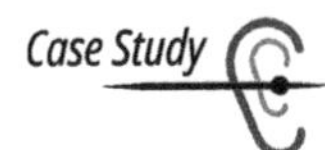

mindset because the mindset acts like a strong foundation. As a doctor, my first step is to strengthen that foundation because once it changes, the subsequent treatment steps become more manageable and easier.

2# My Assurance: Once, a patient came to me, deeply troubled and tired from seeking treatment at many places without finding any relief. He carried with himself reports from about 20 different tests he had undergone. I was surprised and asked, "What is all this?" He explained that he had spent a lot more than he could afford, that is around 1.25 lakh rupees, on these tests, of which 75,000 rupees were borrowed. He mentioned that he neither had access to Employee's State Insurance (ESI) nor did he have a government job; he worked in a private company where he earned a meagre salary of 12,500 rupees per month. Despite all his efforts and expenses, his condition hadn't improved. His story made me very sad. He had reports from five different doctors and yet had no relief from his sufferings. Seeing all this, I felt a deep sense of regret and agony. I felt as if my heart was crying inside, wondering why someone with limited means had to go through such distress—going through so many tests and treatments that drained his resources. It made me wonder how many people like him face similar challenges every day. I assured him that he would get better, and I would treat him. In our first meeting, I focused on boosting his spirits, giving him hope that he would improve, and that there was no need to worry. I tried to change his way of thinking.

3# USA se Aaya Mera Dost (A friend of USA): I remember a patient of mine, Mr. John, from the USA. I vividly recall that he visited India for a business meeting in Delhi, where I was introduced to him by my close friend, Mr. Dinesh. Mr. John had shared his health struggles with Dinesh Ji. Dinesh Ji described me to him as a renowned doctor known worldwide for my generous service, someone who believes in the miracle of healing.

Dinesh Ji went on to say, "I understand that you must have consulted numerous doctors globally, highly knowledgeable and skilled in their field. However, sometimes certain situations go beyond their expertise. That's when we should seek individuals who possess not only knowledge but also divine grace, those who can help people overcome any challenge. Doctor M K Gupta is one such individual", and Dinesh Ji insisted that he should meet me.

With Dinesh Ji's reference, Mr. John came to see me, and it was our first meeting. During our conversation, he seemed discouraged and resigned to living with his illness, convinced that it could not be cured. He had mentally accepted his illness as a constant companion. I explained to him that his

 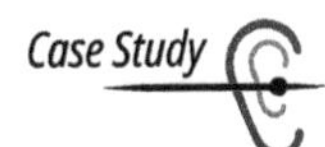

subconscious mind had accepted this illness as a friend, albeit a wrong one, and as we know, “bad company yields bad results”. I made him realise that this illness could be cured, and he agreed with my guidance. Explaining this to him was not very challenging because deep down, he had some awareness of his subconscious mind but lacked proper guidance. After our initial meeting, he began to feel more at ease and was positive about the outcome of the treatment. In our subsequent meetings, I explained our treatment process, detailing the protocols we follow. I assured him that we had successfully resolved many seemingly impossible cases using these methods, and we would do the same with him.

We commenced his treatment, and within 17 days, he had improved by more than 30%. He felt much better and happier, even reaching out from the USA to express his joy. We continued to stay connected through phone calls. He sent chocolates as a gesture of thanks. I felt proud and content, having made a positive change in his life. I consider this as my true earnings, the passion that drives me to continue helping people.

These were just a few stories from my journey, and many more await to be shared. Each of them has left an indelible mark on my path, shaping my beliefs and practices as a doctor. In the chapters ahead, we'll explore the lessons they've brought to my life as a doctor. These stories are not just about medical cases but about people-individuals who trusted me to be more than a healer of ailments, individuals who sought hope and found it in their darkest hours. With each narrative, we'll explore the power of a positive mindset and its profound impact on the human spirit.

Join me on this magnificent journey, where we'll find out more about the positive reinforcement of our mindset.

My Story

My journey as a doctor is filled with hopes and aspirations – the hopes of my patients that they will get well and my aspiration as a doctor to give them my best. 'My Story' takes you along this path, where I'd like to share a few incidents that fueled my determination.

Beyond Medicine:

Considering Patients as People who need help and not mere Cases:

When I started off with my career, I noticed that the way doctors handled their patients had a lot of impact on the outcome of the treatment. I recall a time when a neighbor's child hurt his ear in an accident. The doctor declared the injury as permanent, and the child would stay deaf throughout his life. In India, people regard doctors as a god, so the parents believed the doctor completely. This event left a huge impact on me.

During my studies, I started seeing more cases where doctors and the community said that certain treatments were impossible or very hard, costing a lot with no guarantee of success. However, my determination to help, along with blessings from the almighty, compelled me to undertake these challenging cases. I managed to help many such patients who had lost hope.

So, this realization dawned on me early–that people go to a doctor with a lot of hope and trust, believing that the doctor will help them recover from their illness. Making these hopes come true is what motivates me. Many patients have told me that I'm different from other doctors they've seen. They appreciate the way I treat them, not just as patients, but as regular people. They often say, 'You don't treat us like mere patients; you treat us like we matter.' They also mention that I focus not only on their illness but also on their way of thinking. I believe that how we think is really important. When we work on having a more positive mindset, it helps us overcome tough situations and illnesses. When we work on changing our mindset, we often see a positive change in our actions. We start looking at things more positively, which makes us feel better and helps us balance our life. It also gives us the motivation to get better.

The feedback I receive from patients and our community is overwhelming and touches me deeply. It's the emotional fuel that acts as the driving force to continue my passion burning brightly. I stand tall with pride, knowing that I can be a guiding light for those struggling with these difficulties.

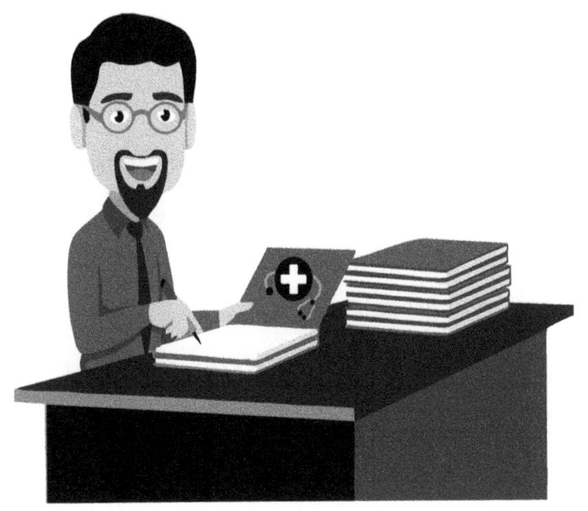

About Author

I am Dr. Manoj Kumar Gupta, the Chief Consultant in the field of Ear, Nose, and Throat (ENT) and the founder Director of Satkriti Hospitals Private Limited. My educational journey includes obtaining an MBBS degree from Silchar Medical College in 1999, followed by an M.S. (ENT) degree from Assam Medical College, Dibrugarh in 2004. Subsequently, I had the privilege of working at AIIMS, New Delhi, where I worked with Prof. R.C. Deka, the esteemed Director of AIIMS. During this time, I engaged in specialized Short Term Training in ENT and also contributed as a Senior Research Fellow on a significant WHO Project.

Throughout my career, I have treated more than 10 Lakhs patients and successfully performed over 10,000 surgeries, including 100,000+ ENT procedures. I've also organized more than 500 camps to provide medical assistance to those in need.

When I was working at AIIMS, I noticed something important. A lot of patients, especially from places like Uttar Pradesh and Bihar, were coming to the hospital for treatment, even for small problems like fungal infections and ear discharge. What caught my attention was that these patients were facing a lot of difficulties. You see, they didn't have good ENT hospitals nearby for these problems, so they had to travel all the way to Delhi.

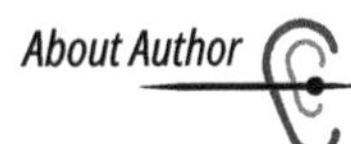

Now, the problem was that many of these patients didn't have much money. Traveling to Delhi and staying there for treatment cost them a lot. And it wasn't just about money. They also had to take time off from their jobs, which meant they couldn't earn during that time. On top of that, they often had to bring family members along to help them, which added even more to their expenses.

Imagine all of these challenges together – the money they had to spend, the time away from work, and the extra costs for their family to come along. It created a big burden for these patients, who were already dealing with health issues. This situation made me realize that there was a need for better healthcare facilities closer to their homes.

Realizing how important it was, I decided to take action. I decided to start a special ENT hospital in Varanasi & Poorvanchal. Even though I didn't earn a lot (only around 12,000 to 15,000 rupees each month), I started saving a little bit of money every month – sometimes just 500 or 1000 rupees. It might not seem like a lot, but over time, these small savings added up. By the time 2012 came, my wife, Dr. Priyanka, and I had saved a good amount – around 8 lakhs.

With this money as our starting point, we came back to Varanasi with a big dream in our hearts. Our dream was to start a healthcare project that could help people in Purvanchal. We wanted to provide them with good medical care right in their own area, so they wouldn't have to go far for treatment. And that's how our journey began.

When we reached Varanasi with 8 lakhs in our bank account, we felt a sense of happiness. But there were challenges like not enough electricity, so we spent around 1.5 lakhs on a Kirloskar genset. We also got a Wagon R car for 4 lakhs and a Honda bike for 0.5 lakhs to solve transportation issues. These things helped us get ready for what was coming. With 2 lakhs left, we started working on turning our home into a clinic, which took about two months.

Since we didn't have a way to earn money immediately, I thought about working in a hospital to make some money. However, my experience in the ENT departments of various hospitals in Varanasi wasn't satisfying. Still, my focus remained on helping patients. So, I took positions in charitable hospitals like RKM, Marwari Hospital, Janta Hospital, and Bunkar. Even though I wasn't paid for these roles, being able to treat patients brought me immense happiness. The appreciation and kindness from patients helped us build strong bonds in a short time.

Finally, on September 2, 2012, we laid the foundation of Satkriti ENT & Sugar Hospital. The rest, as they say, is history.

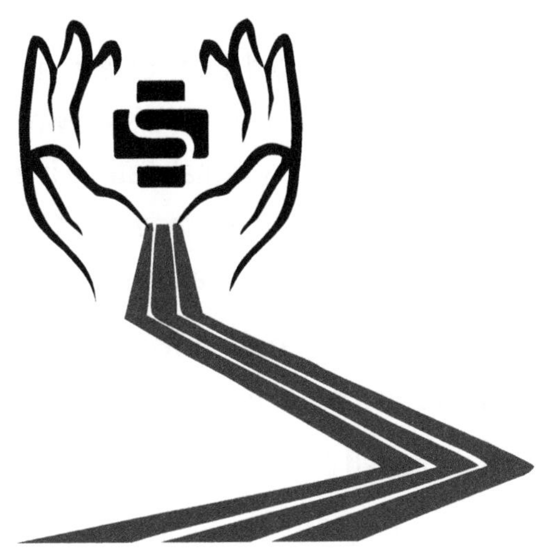

Satkriti Hospital: A Journey of Noble Healing

Satkriti Hospitals Private Limited gets its name from the Sanskrit word "Satkriti", which means "Noble Work" or "Treating With Respect". This name perfectly captures the hospital's main goal – to care for people and help them feel better. Dr. Manoj Kumar Gupta, a respected expert in the field of ENT, and Dr. Priyanka, started the hospital in 2012. It's located in the center of the city and focuses on treating ear, nose, and throat problems as well as diabetes.

Satkriti Hospital is a fully equipped and authorized place where you can get advanced care for ear, nose, and throat (ENT) problems as well as diabetes. It's known as the top ENT Hospital in Varanasi and Purvanchal. Satkriti is always working hard to create improved solutions for various ENT and diabetic issues, aiming to make people healthier and happier.

Satkriti Hospital has done many things for the first time in the area:

- First dedicated ENT hospital in Purvanchal/Varanasi
- First and only ENT Hospital of Varanasi with NABH Accreditation
- First ENT Hospital of this region to launch Ayushman Bharat services
- Pioneered OAE (Otoacoustic Emission) screening for newborns to detect hearing loss
- Introduced endoscopic examination for ENT patients

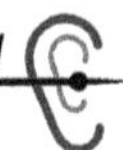

- Pioneered Coblation Surgery in the region
- Established the first Vertigo Lab for patients with dizziness
- First private hospital in Uttar Pradesh to install Zeiss Extaro 300 microscope with integrated camera
- First in the region to initiate modular operation theaters
- First and only ENT Hospital of Varanasi and Poorvanchal to have NABH accreditation.
- Only ENT Hospital in Varanasi Empanelled for ADIP CI Scheme of Govt. of India.

Satkriti Hospitals Private Limited is determined to be the best place for healthcare. It comes from a long history of wanting to help others, and it's always trying new and smart ways to take care of patients. The hospital focuses on making ears, nose, throat (ENT), and diabetes better. With each move forward, we are aiming to make people healthier and happier. Our goal is to bring new ideas and good health to the people we take care of, making their future brighter.

Vision : Freedom from Deafness To make India Free from Deafness by 2047

Mission : To be one of the most admired ENT Hospital in Asia by 2030

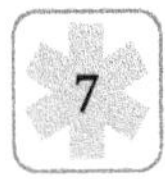

Values :

1# Committed to Heal

2# Patientwell being is our priority

3# Honest and Open Communication with patients and amongst Team Members

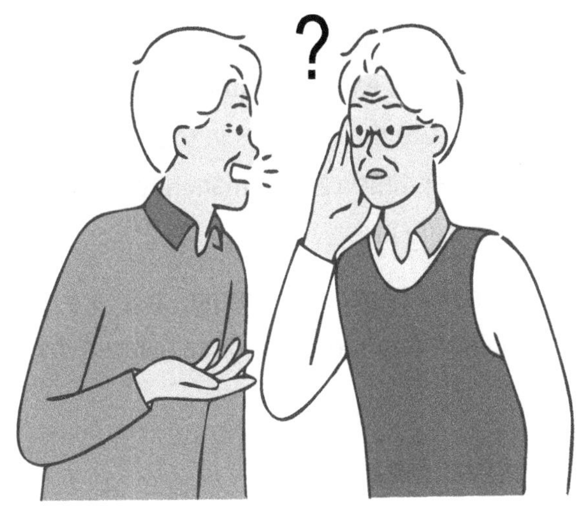

Breaking the Silence: A Closer Look at Deafness

Deafness is a condition where someone can't hear well or might not hear anything at all. This range of hearing problems can be from a bit of trouble hearing to a big issue, affecting one or both ears. It can be something you're born with or something that happens as you grow up due to things like family history, sickness, getting older, loud noises, or other health problems.

How hearing loss occurs:

Hearing loss can occur due to various factors that affect the delicate structures of the ear and the auditory system. The sound vibrates the eardrum and the tiny bones in the ear, which, in turn, vibrate the hair cells in the inner ear. Exposure to loud noises over time can permanently damage the hair cells, causing hearing loss.

The two main types of hearing loss are conductive and sensorineural hearing loss, often caused by different mechanisms:

Conductive Deafness:

This happens when something in the outer or middle part of the ear blocks sounds from going to the inner ear. This could be things like too much earwax, liquid in the ear (like when you have an ear infection), or problems with how the ear is shaped.

Here are some examples that might cause Conductive Deafness:

- **Impacted Wax:** If too much stuff called ear wax builds up in your ear, it can stop sounds from traveling through and make it harder to hear.
- **Ear Infection:** When your ear gets sick, there can be liquid inside the middle of the ear that makes it tricky for sounds to move, so hearing might be tough for a while.
- **Bones in Ear Don't Move Right:** The tiny bones in your ear might not move like they should, and that can make it tricky to hear things (Otosclerosis).
- **Hole in Eardrum:** If there's a hole in your eardrum, it won't work well, and you might not hear things as clearly.
- **Things Stuck in Ear / Foreign Body:** If something gets stuck inside your ear, it can block sounds and make it hard for you to hear.
- **Ear Gets Hurt / Trauma:** If your ear gets hurt, like from a bump or accident, it can make hearing things properly a bit tough.
- **Unusual Things Growing:** Rarely, strange things might grow in your ear and make it harder for sounds to get through.

- **Ear Bones Not Right:** Sometimes, the bones in your ear don't grow the way they're supposed to, and that can make hearing a bit tricky.
- **Sensorineural Deafness:** This kind comes from damage to the inner ear or the nerves that take sound to the brain. It might happen because of getting older, really loud noises, certain medicines, things that are in your family, or other health issues.

A few factors that could result in Sensorineural Deafness include:

- **Getting Older:** As people grow older, their hearing can become less sharp, making it harder to hear things clearly.
- **Loud Noises:** Being around really loud noises, like fireworks or loud music, for a long time can damage your hearing and make it harder to hear well.
- **Certain Medicines:** Some medicines, especially if taken in big amounts, can harm the tiny hair cells in your ears that help you hear.
- **Family History:** If others in your family also have trouble hearing, it could be because of something that's passed down in your genes.

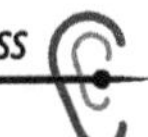

- **Health Issues:** Some health problems, like diabetes or heart conditions, can also affect your hearing over time.
- **Unknown:** Sudden SNHL

Levels of Hearing Loss:

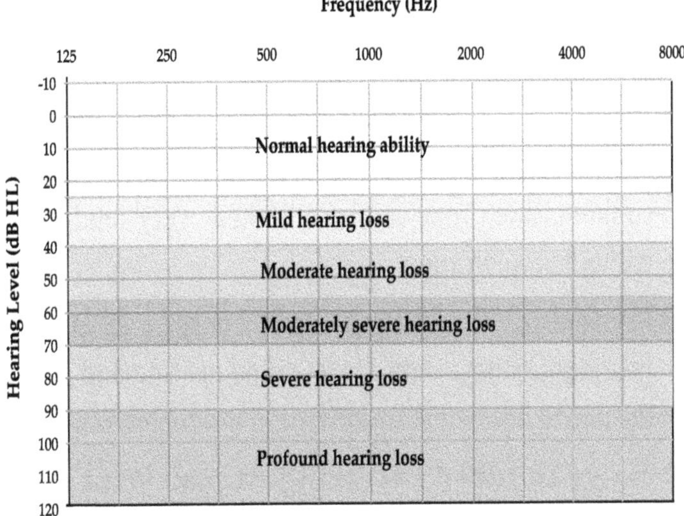

The level of hearing loss refers to how much someone's ability to hear has been affected. It's usually categorized into different degrees based on the severity of the impairment:

1# Mild Hearing Loss: People with mild hearing loss may have difficulty hearing soft sounds or distant speech. They might miss certain words or parts of conversations, especially in noisy environments.

2# **Moderate Hearing Loss:** Those with moderate hearing loss struggle to hear normal conversations without the help of hearing aids. They might miss a lot of what's said, particularly in noisy situations.

3# **Moderately Severe Hearing Loss:** People with moderately severe hearing loss have even more difficulty hearing and understanding speech, especially in group settings or when not using hearing aids.

4# **Severe Hearing Loss:** Individuals with severe hearing loss may rely heavily on lip-reading or sign language to communicate. They might only hear very loud sounds without amplification.

5# **Profound Hearing Loss:** Those with profound hearing loss have extremely limited hearing and may not be able to hear most sounds, even at very high volumes.

6# **Noise-Induced Hearing Loss:** Noise-induced hearing loss (NIHL) is a type of hearing loss that is caused by exposure to loud noise. The loud noise damages the hair cells in the inner ear, which are responsible for hearing. NIHL can be permanent and can lead to difficulty hearing, ringing in the ears (tinnitus), and difficulty understanding speech.

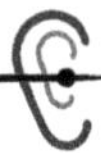

The level of hearing loss affects how well someone can communicate and engage with their environment. It's important to get a proper evaluation from a healthcare professional if you suspect any degree of hearing loss.

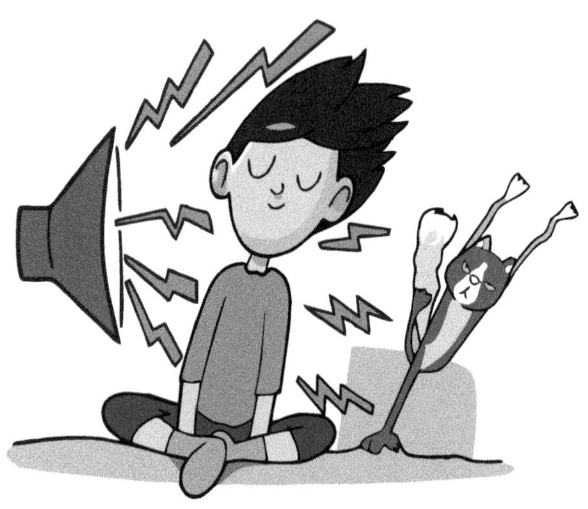

How Loud is too Loud?

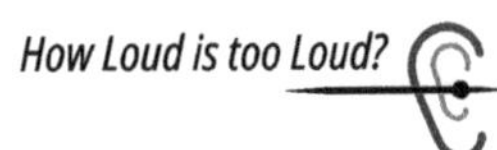

Sound is all around us, shaping our experiences and connecting us to the world. But not all sounds are good for our ears. This chapter delves into the concept of safe listening and uncovers how to distinguish between enjoyable sound and potentially harmful noise. Let's explore this further:

Understanding Decibels: To navigate the realm of sound, we first need to understand a unit called decibels (dB). Decibels measure the loudness of sound. As we explore everyday sounds, we'll learn about the decibel levels of a whisper, normal conversation, music, traffic, and even fireworks.

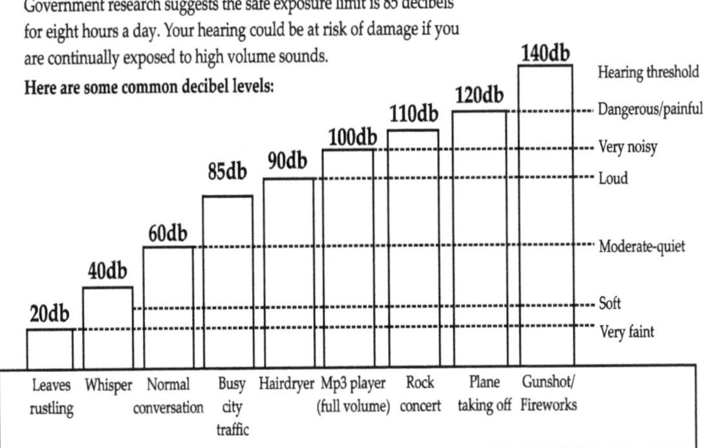

When Sound Becomes Noise:

While some sounds are soothing, others can be damaging. We'll explore how sounds become noise when they reach high decibel levels. Discover what happens inside our ears when exposed to excessive noise and how it can lead to hearing problems over time.

The Risks of Loud Environments:

From concerts to construction sites, our surroundings can often be quite noisy. This section delves into the risks associated with prolonged exposure to loud environments. We'll look at occupations and activities that may put people at a higher risk of hearing damage.

Personal Audio Devices:

In the digital age, personal audio devices have become a constant companion. But cranking up the volume too high can lead to serious consequences. This book explores the safe use of headphones and earbuds to prevent unnecessary harm to our hearing.

Protecting Our Ears:

Prevention is key. We'll discuss practical ways in the upcoming chapters to protect our ears from loud noises, including using earplugs, taking listening breaks, and maintaining a safe distance from noisy sources.

Guidelines for Safe Listening:

To enjoy life without compromising our hearing, we'll outline guidelines for safe listening. This includes recommendations for the volume settings on personal devices, strategies for attending loud events, and fostering awareness among friends and family.

Conclusion:

In a world filled with sounds both beautiful and potentially harmful, learning how loud is too loud becomes essential. By understanding decibels, recognizing noisy environments, and adopting safe listening habits, we can preserve our hearing and continue to savor the symphony of life.

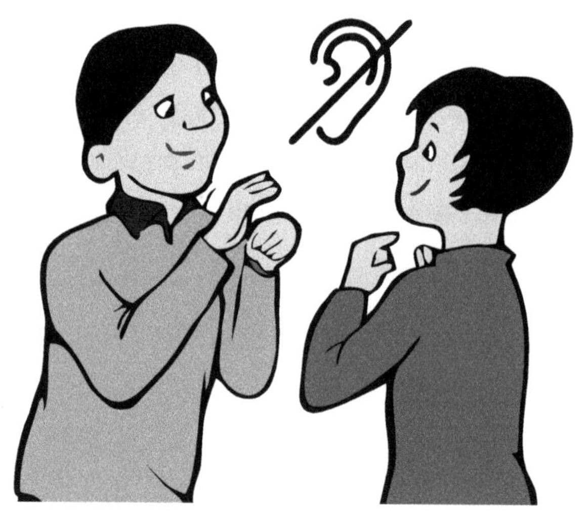

Being Aware: Deafness

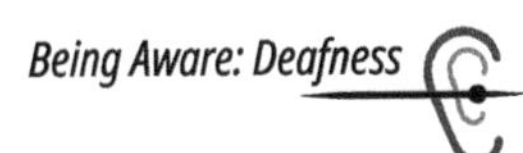

Deafness can change how we talk with others, make friends, and enjoy life. People who can't hear well might use different ways to chat, like using special signs with their hands, reading lips, writing things down, or using tools to help them listen better, like special ear devices.

Being aware of deafness is really important because it helps us understand how it happens, how to prevent it, and how to help people who are dealing with it. When we know about deafness, we can do things to prevent it, like being careful around loud noises that can hurt our ears.

When we're aware, we can also support people who are already having trouble hearing. We can learn how to communicate with them better, and we can make sure they get the right help, like using special devices that make sounds clearer.

So, being aware about deafness isn't just good for people who have hearing problems, it's good for all of us. It makes us better at taking care of our ears and being kind to others who might be going through a tough time with their hearing.

Awareness holds the answer. But why is awareness so important?

Well, consider this: almost half of all cases of deafness can actually be prevented. That's right, 50% of hearing problems can be stopped from happening. And even when hearing issues can't be stopped, about 30% of them can be helped with special devices.

So, let's put it together: if we know more and spread the word, we can prevent a big part—about 80%—of hearing problems.

Here's a fact that really drives it home: when it comes to hearing loss caused by loud noises, we can totally stop it from happening. It's 100% preventable. But if someone gets this kind of hearing loss, it sticks around for life.

That's why awareness matters so much. It's not just about knowing, it's about changing lives.

Here are some surprising facts about hearing loss:

- Around 1.5 billion people worldwide, which is about 20% of the global population, are dealing with hearing problems.
- Most of these people, around 1.16 billion, have a mild hearing loss .

- Almost 470 million people, which is around 5.5% of the world's population, have more serious hearing issues. If they don't get help, it might affect their daily life.
- Around 400 million people have hearing problems that are somewhere between a bit of trouble and a lot of trouble.
- There are about 30 million people who can't hear at all in both of their ears.
- Nowadays, 1 out of every 5 people around the world has hearing problems.
- But by the year 2050, it's predicted that 1 out of every 4 people might have issues with their hearing.
- Most of the people who have trouble hearing, almost 80% of them, live in countries where money is limited.
- In the year 2019, 1.5 billion people had hearing problems, but it's expected to be 1.9 billion by 2030, 2.2 billion by 2040, and 2.5 billion by 2050.
- In India, about 75 million people (7.5 crore) have significant hearing problems.
- Hearing problems are the second most common reason people have trouble with things. The biggest reason is not being able to sense things properly.

- Every day, about 300 babies are born with trouble hearing. That's around 1 lakh babies every year.
- About 4 out of every 1000 children can't hear well, and their hearing problems are pretty serious.

More and more people are having trouble with their hearing, and it's important to think about this seriously. The number of people who can't hear well is going up. This means that lots of people are having a hard time understanding sounds and talking with others.

This is something we shouldn't ignore. As the world changes and it gets noisier around us, more people are being around things that can hurt their hearing. If we don't do something about it, hearing problems can really change how someone lives every day. They might have trouble talking to people, enjoying music, being part of fun activities, or doing well in school or work. Hearing loss greatly affects the quality of life, and individuals suffering from it are at a higher risk of developing depression and other mental health issues.

Seeing that more people are having hearing problems shows us that we need to know more about it, help early on, and have things that can make a difference. If we take hearing problems seriously and try to stop them from happening, we can make a world where everyone can talk and listen clearly and have a good time.

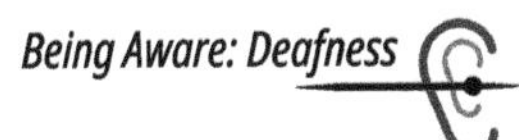

To help with deafness, it depends on what's causing it and how serious it is. Talking to doctors, hearing experts, and specialists can help find the best way to make things better for each person.

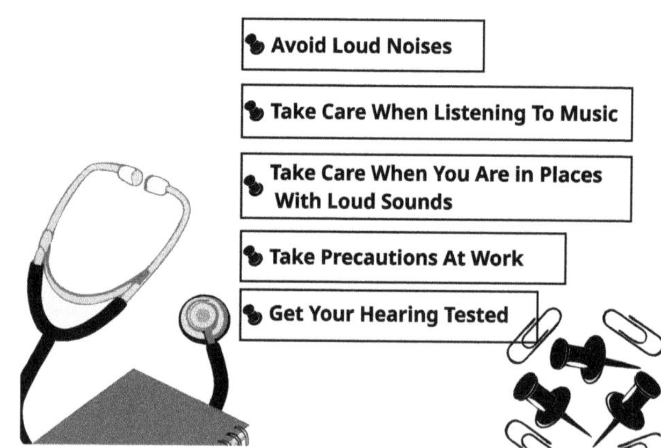

5 Ways to Prevent Hearing Loss Due to Exposure to Loud Noise

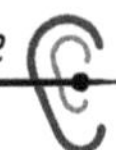

The way hearing loss happens is like a big puzzle with different pieces. Some parts are things we can't control and are linked to getting older. This means that as we age, our ability to hear can decrease naturally. But there's another part related to how loud noises affect our hearing, and this part can be prevented. If we're exposed to really loud sounds for a long time, like when there's a lot of noise around us, it can hurt our ears and make us lose our ability to hear well. The good news is that we can do things to avoid this kind of hearing loss. Whether we're young and full of energy or older and experienced, making sure we don't damage our hearing is really important. The more years go by and the more things we go through, the clearer it becomes that small and easy steps can prevent big and irreversible problems with our hearing. Imagine life's energy and excitement as a beautiful song, and these steps as the steady beat that keeps the rhythm going, connecting all generations and keeping our hearing safe.

Hearing loss cannot always be prevented – sometimes it's just part of getting older. But hearing loss due to exposure to loud noises is completely avoidable. There are some simple things you can do to help stop loud noises from permanently damaging your hearing, no matter how old you are.

Here are the 5 Effective Ways to Protect Your Hearing, from the Dangers of Loud Noise:

1# Avoid Loud Noises

We all know that loud noises can hurt our ears, but did you know there's a way to make sure they don't damage our hearing? The best thing we can do is to stay away from really loud sounds as much as possible. But how do we know if a sound is too loud? Well, there are some signs to watch out for.

Imagine you're talking to a friend. If you have to shout to hear each other, the noise around you might be too loud. Or if you can't understand what people nearby are saying because of the noise, that's another hint. And if a noise hurts your ears, that's a big sign that it's too loud. Even after the noise stops, if your ears ring or everything sounds muffled, it means your ears were exposed to too much noise.

Now, sounds are measured using something called decibels (dB). The higher the number, the louder the sound. Any sound over 85 dB can be harmful, especially if we're around it for a long time. Here are some examples to help you understand:

When someone whispers, it's about 30 dB.

Talking normally is around 60 dB.

When there's lots of traffic, it's 70-85 dB.

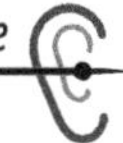

A motorcycle can be 90 dB.

If you listen to music super loud through headphones, it can reach 100-120 dB.

A plane taking off is about 120 dB.

We can even use special apps on our phones to measure how loud things are. Just make sure the app is set up correctly to get the right information.

By knowing all this, we can be in control of our hearing health. Remember, if something is really loud and it hurts your ears or makes them ring, it's a sign to give your ears a break. Taking care of our ears means we can enjoy all the sounds around us without worrying about hurting our hearing.

2# Take Care When Listening To Music

Did you know that listening to super loud music with earphones or headphones can be really bad for your ears? But don't worry, there are things you can do to keep your hearing safe:

- **Use Special Earphones or Headphones:** Instead of making the music louder to block outside noises, you can use special noise-cancelling earphones or headphones. This way, you can enjoy your music without needing to turn up the volume.

- **Make the Volume Just Right:** Adjust the volume to a level where you can hear your music comfortably. It's important not to make it too loud.
- **Keep the Volume Low:** Try not to turn the volume up past 60% of the highest level. Some devices can even help you set a limit so it doesn't get too loud.
- **Take Breaks:** If you wear earphones or headphones for more than an hour, it can make your ears tired. So, remember to take a break for at least 5 minutes every hour.
- **Lower the Volume a Little:** Even making the volume a bit lower can really help prevent any harm to your hearing.

By following these steps, you can enjoy your music and also make sure your ears stay healthy. Just remember, these simple things can do a lot to keep your ears safe and sound.

3# Take Care When You Are in Places With Loud Sounds

When you're in places with loud sounds, like nightclubs, concerts, or sports events, you can do some things to keep your hearing safe:

- **Step Away from Loud Sounds:** If there are really loud speakers or noises, try to move away from them. This can help protect your ears.

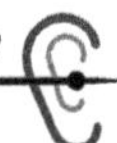

- **Give Your Ears Breaks:** Every 15 minutes or so, try to take a little break from the loud noises. This gives your ears a chance to rest.
- **Let Your Ears Rest:** After being around lots of loud noise, it's good to give your ears about 18 hours to rest and recover.
- **Use Earplugs:** You can wear special earplugs that musicians use. They don't make everything sound muffled, but they do lower the loudness of the music.

By doing these things, you can have fun in loud places and still make sure your ears stay healthy. It's like giving your ears a shield to keep them safe from the noise.

4# Take Precautions At Work

When your job has really loud sounds, it's a good idea to talk to the important people at your workplace, like the Human Resources (HR) folks or the Occupational Health Manager. They can help you avoid loud noise because it's their job to keep you safe. Here are some things they can do, such as:

- **Using Quieter Equipment:** If possible, they can switch to equipment that doesn't make as much noise.
- **Limiting Exposure:** Your employer can make sure you're not around loud noises for too long at a time.

- **Providing Ear Protection:** They might give you special things to wear on your ears, like earmuffs or earplugs, to keep your hearing safe.

Remember, if you're given any ear protection, make sure to wear it. Your hearing is important, and these steps can help you keep it safe while you work.

5# Get Your Hearing Tested

If you feel like your hearing is not as good as before, it's a good idea to get a hearing test quickly. The earlier you know about hearing problems, the quicker you can get help. If you're in jobs or activities where loud noises happen a lot, like if you're a musician or work in noisy places, you might want to check your hearing regularly, maybe once a year. This way, you can stay on top of things and make sure your ears are doing well.

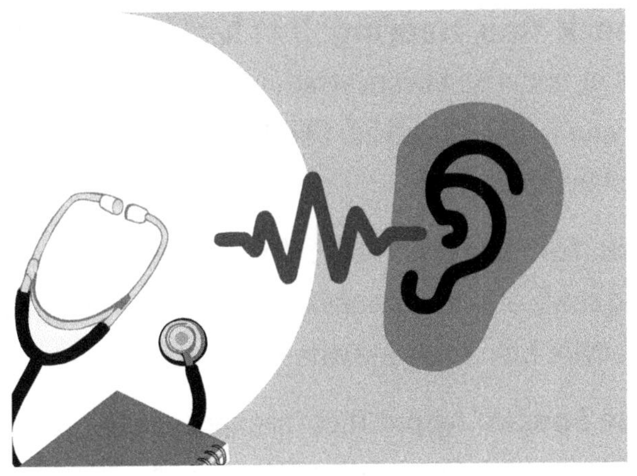

Tips for Safe and Better Hearing

Hear WHO:

If you really like listening to music often, it's really important to take care of your ears. Here are some things you can do to keep your ears safe and healthy:

Pay Attention to Warning Signs: If you notice anything strange with your hearing, it's a big deal. If your ears keep ringing all the time and it doesn't stop, it's a good idea to talk to a doctor.

Check Your Hearing: If it's hard for you to hear high sounds or understand conversations, it might be a good idea to get your hearing checked. Checking regularly can help find any problems early.

Ask for Expert Help: If you have trouble during a hearing check or see any signs of hearing loss, it's a good idea to get advice from someone who knows about ears.

Use Special Apps: There are apps you can use to check how well you hear. Some are recommended by health experts like WHO.

These things are super important, especially when you look at how many people have hearing problems all over the world:

- More than 1 billion young people might have hearing problems because they listen to things too loudly.
- More than 43 million people between 12 and 35 years old can't hear well.
- Many young people in rich countries have issues with hearing:
- Almost half listen to music way too loud on things like MP3 players and phones.
- About 40% are around really loud sounds at places like clubs, bars, and sports events.

By being careful and doing these things, you can enjoy music and all the sounds in life while making sure your ears stay healthy. Remember, taking care of your hearing is like giving your ears a big hug!

Yoga: A Boost for Your Hearing:

Yoga is a mind-body practice that combines physical postures, breathing exercises, and meditation. It has been shown to have many benefits for overall health and well-being, including improved hearing. One of the important functions that we tend to ignore when we think of exercising is hearing. But it is time that one considers taking care of one of the most important organs for the body- ears. Yoga can be one form of effective exercising that can treat various ear problems and progressive hearing loss.

Some of the ways that yoga can help to improve hearing include:

1# **Reducing Stress:** Yoga helps to reduce stress levels, which can indirectly benefit hearing. High stress levels can impact various aspects of health, including hearing health.

2# **Enhancing Blood Circulation:** Certain yoga poses and exercises can improve blood circulation throughout the body, including the ears. Better blood flow can promote healthier ear function.

3# **Relaxation Techniques:** Yoga often incorporates relaxation techniques such as deep breathing and meditation. These practices can help relax the muscles in the ears and promote a sense of calm, which can be beneficial for hearing health.

4# **Improving Posture:** Some yoga poses focus on improving posture. Good posture can help ensure that the structures related to hearing, like the inner ear, are in their optimal position for proper functioning.

5# Strengthening Neck and Shoulder Muscles: Yoga exercises that target neck and shoulder muscles can indirectly support better hearing. Tension in these areas can impact blood flow to the ears and contribute to hearing issues.

6# Boosting Mind-Body Connection: Practicing yoga encourages mindfulness and better awareness of the body. This connection can help you notice any changes in your hearing or overall health more quickly.

7# Promoting General Well-being: Yoga is linked to better overall health, which can have positive effects on various bodily systems, including the ears.

Yoga postures with deep breathing exercises increase oxygen rich blood flow to the ear area. Stretching, muscle relaxation, and deep breathing techniques performed under yoga have a positive impact on heart, blood circulation and blood pressure. A good blood supply to the ears improves the functioning of nerves. An increase of blood supply takes out the toxins from the infected ear and helps to reduce ear infection and ear pain as well.

Presented below is a Yoga Chart featuring yoga postures aimed at promoting better hearing:

Yoga Postures	How to do it
1. Bhramari Pranayama	Sit comfortably, close your eyes, and take a deep breath in. As you exhale, make a humming sound like a bee. This practice helps calm the mind, reduce stress, and improve blood circulation, which can indirectly support auditory health.
2. Bhujangasana	Bhujangasana, or Cobra Pose, involves lying on your stomach, lifting your chest while keeping your lower body grounded, and stretching your arms. This pose enhances blood circulation to the head and neck, supplying more oxygen to the auditory system.
3. Matsyasana	Practicing Fish Pose stretches the neck and throat region, which could potentially support healthy circulation in the auditory system.
4. Ustrasana	Ustrasana, or Camel Pose, involves kneeling, arching your back, and reaching for your heels or ankles while keeping your hips forward. This pose enhances blood circulation to the head and neck, delivering vital nutrients and oxygen to the auditory system.

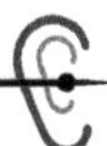

5. Tadasana	Tadasana, or Mountain Pose, involves standing with feet together, lengthening the spine, and relaxing the shoulders. This pose promotes proper posture and alignment, indirectly benefiting the auditory system by enhancing circulation to the head and neck.
6. Vajrasana	Vajrasana, or Thunderbolt Pose, involves kneeling with knees together and sitting back on your heels. This pose aids digestion, indirectly contributing to overall well-being which can impact auditory health.
7. Trikonasana	Trikonasana, or Triangle Pose, involves standing with feet apart, reaching and extending the torso while one arm points downward and the other extends upward. Trikonasana's stretching and alignment-improving qualities also contribute to overall well-being, potentially aiding in better hearing function.

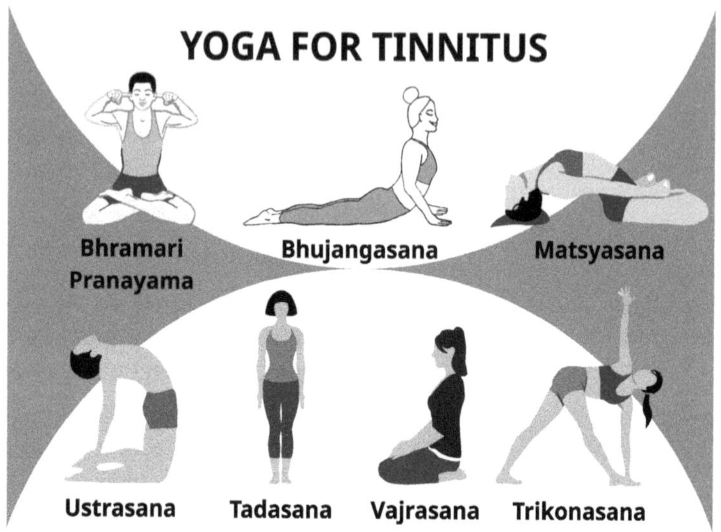

While yoga can contribute to better hearing, it's important to remember that hearing health involves multiple factors. If you have concerns about your hearing, it's advisable to consult a healthcare professional or an audiologist for proper evaluation and guidance. There are many different yoga poses that can be beneficial for hearing such as Bhramari Pranayama, Shunya Mudra, Greeva Chalan, Bhujangasana, Urdhva Dhanurasana, Surya Namaskar, etc.

If you are interested in trying yoga for better hearing, it is important to start slowly and gradually increase the intensity of your practice. It is also important to consult with your doctor before starting any new exercise program, especially if you have any underlying health conditions.

Here are some additional tips for practicing yoga for better hearing:

- Find a qualified yoga instructor who can help you to choose the right poses for your needs.
- Practice yoga regularly, at least 3-4 times per week.
- Focus on your breath during your yoga practice.
- Be patient and consistent with your practice. It may take some time to see results.

Yoga is a safe and effective way to improve hearing. If you are looking for a natural way to improve your hearing, yoga is a good option to consider.

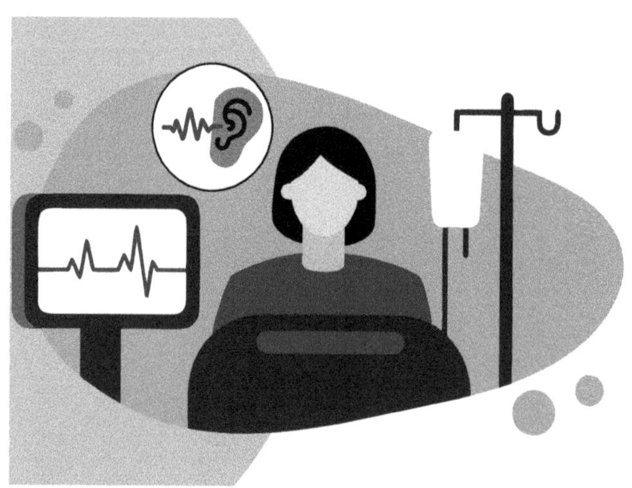

Sudden Hearing Loss: A Critical Medical Emergency

Imagine waking up one day and the world around you goes quiet. Sudden hearing loss can happen unexpectedly, leaving you worried and unsure. This chapter is here to help you understand why fast action is important when you experience sudden hearing loss. We'll talk about what might cause it, how doctors figure it out, and why you should get help right away.

Have you ever thought about how you'd feel if you couldn't hear anymore? Sudden hearing loss doesn't happen to everyone, but it can happen suddenly and make you feel really scared. Approximately one out of every 5,000 adults experiences sudden-onset hearing loss annually, although this number might be much higher due to cases that remain unreported and undiagnosed.

Studies have shown that if an intratympanic injection is administered within the first 48 hours of symptom onset, the chances of successful recovery can soar to nearly 90%. This is why it's very important to see a doctor or go to the hospital as soon as you realize your hearing is gone. The first 48 hours are considered the Golden Period, and if treated promptly, hearing loss may be reversible.

When your hearing disappears all of a sudden, you might feel like something in your ear "popped" or that your ear is full. You could also hear ringing sounds that won't go away. These are signs that tell you something isn't right, and you should get help quickly.

Finding out why sudden hearing loss happens is not easy. The reason behind it is unclear, and while many theories support viral and upper respiratory tract infection (URTI) involvement, none have been proven. Due to its sudden onset and the various potential causes, doctors find it challenging to understand.

Sudden hearing loss is a big deal and needs fast action. By learning about what it is and why you should get help quickly, you'll know how to take care of your hearing and make sure you get the best chance to hear well again.

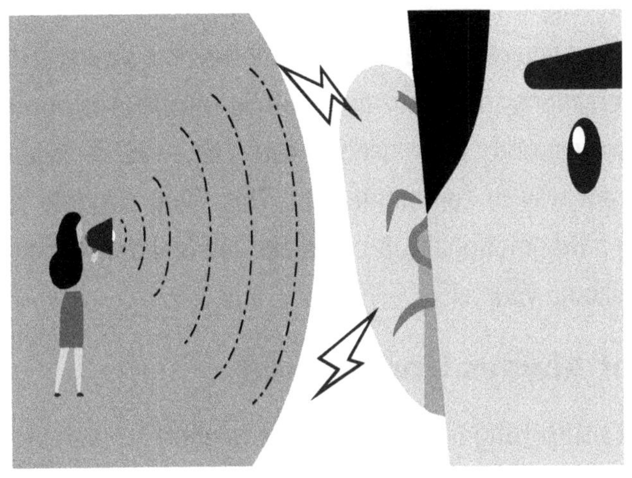

Social Impact of Deafness

Hearing Loss: What You Can't See

Hearing loss is a challenge that's not easy to notice. Its effects are hidden, so it's tough for others to understand how much it can affect someone. Unlike problems you can see, like a broken leg, the impact of hearing loss is not so obvious. People who have it have to deal with it without others really knowing what they're going through.

Living Quietly

When you can't hear well, life can become a quiet struggle. Conversations and music might not be enjoyable anymore. The everyday sounds we're used to can fade away, replaced by a different way of communicating. This silent struggle can be really hard emotionally. It can make you feel down and not so good about yourself.

Not Always Understood

It's surprising that some people might react with laughter instead of understanding when they learn someone has hearing loss. Unlike when someone is blind and people usually feel sorry, hearing loss can sometimes make people laugh or not take it seriously. This adds to the tough feelings that people with hearing loss face.

Feeling Alone, Even with Family

Hearing loss can even cause problems within families. Misunderstandings can happen because of communication gaps. This can create a wall between people with hearing loss and their loved ones. Not being able to join in conversations and activities can lead to a sense of being left out and feeling alone.

Struggling in School

When kids have hearing loss, school can be a real challenge. Understanding lessons, communicating with teachers, and making friends might not be as easy. This can affect their academic performance and their self-confidence.

Why Talking Helps

It's important to talk about the emotional struggles of hearing loss. People who can't hear well often deal with loneliness, worry, and even sadness. Not being able to connect with others like before can make them feel not so good. Getting the right help, like talking to someone who understands, is important to handle these feelings. They are at a higher risk of depression and other mental health issues.

Tough Times for Kids

When hearing loss starts from a young age, it can be even harder. Things like learning to speak and making friends can be tricky. This difficulty can last a long time and affect things like school and jobs when they grow up.

The End Goal

Hearing loss is much more than just missing out on sounds. The struggles that people with hearing loss face are deeper and harder to see. To make a world where everyone feels included, we need to learn more about hearing loss and support each other with kindness and understanding.

It's worth asking: Why do some deaf people become mute?

Deaf people might not use their voices to talk because they've never heard how normal sounds and speech sound. Imagine if you've never heard someone speak or the sound of a bird singing – it would be really hard to know how to make those sounds yourself.

For people who were born deaf, speaking can be quite challenging. They didn't get the chance to learn how to copy the sounds they've never heard. It's like trying to play a song on a piano you've never seen or heard before.

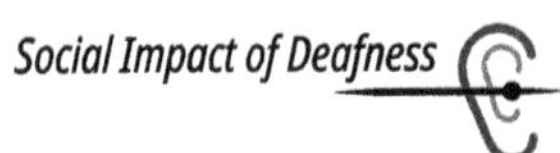

On the other hand, for those who became deaf later in life or during childhood after they've already learned to talk, it might be a bit easier. They remember how sounds and speech work, so even though they can't hear as well anymore, they still have an idea of how to make the right sounds.

In simple words, becoming mute – not using your voice to talk – can happen because understanding how to make sounds when you've never heard them is really tricky. It's like trying to draw a picture with your eyes closed.

HEARING DAY

HEARING DAY

		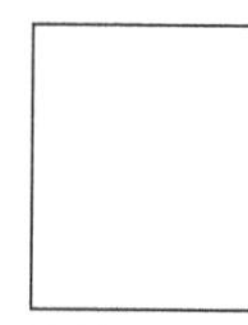	
03 MARCH World Hearing Day	**26 SEPT** Day of Deaf in India	**LAST WEEK OF SEPTEMBER** International Week of Deaf	**2006** National Programme for Prevention and Control of Deafness (NPPCD)

1# World Hearing Day is an annual event held on March 3rd to raise awareness about hearing loss and promote ear health. It's organized by the World Health Organization (WHO) to highlight the importance of taking care of our ears and addressing hearing-related issues.

2# September 26th is observed as "Day of Deaf in India".

3# The International Week of the Deaf is a global observance

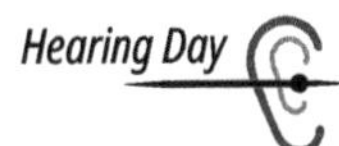

that typically takes place during the last full week of September, leading up to International Day of the Deaf in the last week of September. This week-long event is dedicated to raising awareness about the rights, issues, and achievements of deaf individuals worldwide.

During the International Week of the Deaf, various activities, events, and campaigns are organized to promote deaf culture, sign language, and the empowerment of deaf people. It provides an opportunity to highlight the challenges that deaf individuals face, such as access to education, communication, and social inclusion, and to advocate for their rights and equal opportunities.

4# The National Programme for Prevention and Control of Deafness (NPPCD) was launched in India in 2006. This program is aimed at preventing and controlling hearing loss and deafness at the national level. Its primary focus is on creating awareness about ear health, promoting early detection of hearing problems, providing medical interventions, and improving the overall ear health infrastructure in the country.

Do's and Don'ts While Cleaning Your Ears

Do's:

Clean the Outer Ear: Gently clean the outer part of your ear with a soft washcloth during your regular bath or shower.

Use Warm Water: If you feel the need to clean inside your ears, you can use warm water. Let a few drops of warm water flow into your ear while tilting your head. Then, tilt your head the other way to let the water come out.

Consult a Doctor: If you have excessive earwax or feel discomfort, it's best to consult a doctor. They can advise you on safe ways to remove excess wax or address any issues.

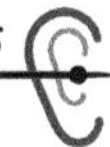

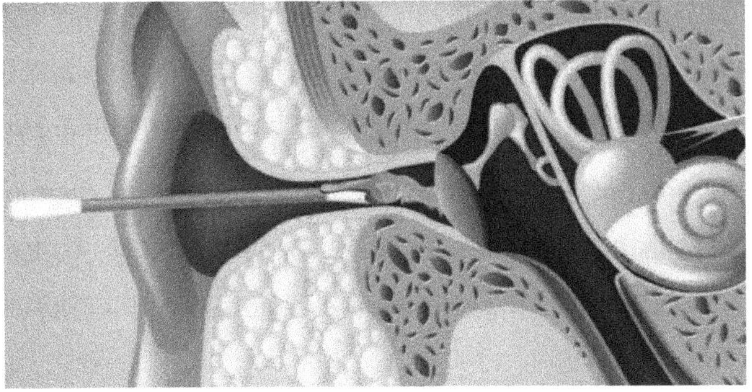

Don'ts:

Insert Objects: Never insert objects like cotton swabs, bobby pins, keys, or any small items into your ears. This can push wax deeper, potentially causing damage or blockages.

Use Q-Tips: Q-Tips or cotton swabs should not be used inside your ear canal. They can push wax further in and even damage the delicate lining of the ear canal.

Aggressive Cleaning: Avoid using forceful methods to clean your ears. This can irritate the ear canal and lead to infections.

Ear Candling: Stay away from ear candling, a method where a hollow cone is placed in the ear and lit. It's not proven to be safe or effective and can be dangerous.

Excess Cleaning: Your ears naturally produce earwax to protect your ear canal. Cleaning too often can disrupt this process and lead to dryness or irritation.

Self-Diagnosis: If you experience pain, hearing loss, or unusual sensations in your ears, don't try to diagnose and treat the issue yourself. It's best to seek professional medical advice.

Remember, your ears are delicate, and gentle cleaning is usually all that's needed. If you're unsure or have concerns, it's always a good idea to consult a healthcare professional for guidance.

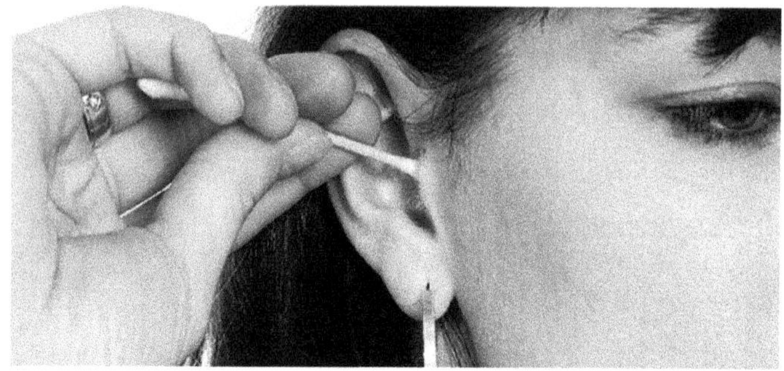

Cotton buds can damage your ear

Frequently Asked Questions (FAQs)

Question 1: Is it possible that I am experiencing hearing loss?

Answer: You might be facing hearing loss if you:

1# Frequently request others to repeat themselves.

2# Increase the volume of the radio or television.

3# Struggle to follow conversations in noisy environments.

4# Find it challenging to understand phone conversations.

5# Experience a ringing sensation in the ear (tinnitus).

6# Encounter difficulty hearing sounds like doorbell alarms or telephone rings.

7# Receive feedback from others that you speak loudly.

Question 2: Why is early diagnosis important?

Answer: Detecting significant hearing loss early is crucial, as not catching it in time can result in delays in speech and language development. Identifying hearing loss early and providing proper care improves a child's speech, language, and education, helping them reach their full potential.

Did you know? Around 90% of hearing-impaired children worldwide live in countries where resources are limited, making it challenging to carry out newborn hearing screening.

Question 3: What is the difference between Earphones and Headphones?

Answer: Earphones, also called earbuds, are tinier and usually made from materials like silicone or hard plastic. They fit comfortably into your ear canal. Because of their design, earphones push the sound really close to your eardrum. This can make the sound too loud and harm your hearing.

On the other hand, headphones cover your whole ear. They're bigger and keep out extra noise from around you. This can be helpful if you're in a noisy place.

Remember the 60:60 Rule:

Here's a helpful rule: Keep the volume of your device around 60% of its loudest for up to 60 minutes. Then give your ears a break for 10 minutes. This way, you take care of your ears and help protect your hearing.

Question 4: Is deafness a disability?

Answer: Deafness is considered a disability in terms of its impact on hearing, communication, and social interactions. However, many deaf individuals lead fulfilling lives and contribute to society in various ways.

Question 5: Can deaf people communicate?

Answer: Yes, deaf people can communicate using various methods, including sign language, lip reading, writing, and using assistive devices like hearing aids and cochlear implants.

Question 6: What is sign language?

Answer: Sign language is a visual way of communicating using hand gestures, facial expressions, and body movements. Different countries have their own sign languages.

Question 7: What is Tinnitus?

Answer: Tinnitus is a sound that comes from within the ear, rather than an outside source. It is not clear why people develop tinnitus, but it often occurs with hearing loss.

People can experience tinnitus in different ways. People may hear buzzing, humming, grinding or whistling. These sounds can be constant or irregular.

Question 8: Can ear candles remove earwax?

Answer: Ear candles are not safe or effective for removing earwax. Consult a healthcare professional for proper earwax removal.

Question 9: Can hearing loss impact mental health?

Answer: Yes, untreated hearing loss can lead to feelings of isolation, depression, and cognitive decline. Treating hearing loss can improve overall well-being.

Question 10: Can certain medical conditions contribute to hearing loss?

Answer: Yes, conditions like diabetes, cardiovascular issues, and autoimmune disorders can affect hearing. Managing these conditions may help prevent hearing loss.

MYTHS AND FACTS

1# MYTH:

Hearing aids will restore my hearing to normal, just like eyeglasses can restore vision to "20/20".

FACT: Hearing aids do not restore hearing to a "normal" state or "cure" hearing loss. Similar to eyeglasses, hearing aids offer benefits by improving hearing and listening abilities, enhancing quality of life. However, hearing aids have limitations. Even individuals with normal hearing experience difficulty hearing in noisy environments. The human ear is a complex system with thousands of nerve endings, making it difficult for a hearing aid to replicate the precision of a normal ear.

2# MYTH:

A hearing aid will damage my hearing.

FACT: A properly fitted, well-maintained, and correctly worn hearing aid will not damage your hearing. The hearing aid is designed to cater to your specific hearing loss.

3# MYTH:

The smaller hearing aids are the best hearing aids.

FACT: There are various styles of hearing aids, all of which are "state-of-the-art". What truly matters is that a hearing aid is tailored to your specific hearing loss and listening requirements. Just because a friend or relative uses a particular hearing aid style doesn't mean it's the best choice for you. Their chosen style might not be suitable for your hearing loss or listening needs. Additionally, not everyone can comfortably use smaller hearing aids.

4# MYTH:

Hearing aids will fix all my communication problems.

FACT: Hearing aids can be very helpful, but there might still be challenges in certain noisy environments, like crowds and restaurants. It's important to note that even individuals with normal hearing struggle to hear well in these settings.

Hearing aids are not flawless, but they do assist you in:

- Hearing softer sounds
- Improving hearing in background noise (like in a cafeteria)
- Enhancing speech understanding

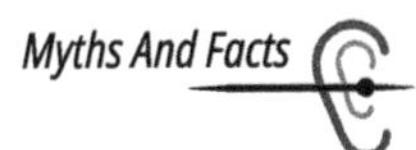

In addition to wearing hearing aids, we recommend using effective listening strategies such as maintaining eye contact with the speaker and reducing the distance between you and the speaker.

5# MYTH:

I will like my new hearing aids the day I get them.

FACT: You might not immediately like your new hearing aids when you first wear them. Hearing aids help you hear many sounds you haven't heard in a while. At first, some noises might seem loud, and even your own voice could sound different. It could take a few weeks to get used to them. It's a good idea to start using them when you're relaxed, like at home watching TV or talking with just one person in the room. Give yourself time to adjust to them.

6# MYTH:

My hearing will get worse because my ears will depend on the hearing aids.

FACT: Wearing a properly fitted hearing aid will not make your hearing worse. Hearing aids help your ears hear sounds that might not be heard without them. When you don't use a hearing aid, your ears miss out on these sounds, and your brain forgets what they were like. It's important to keep your ears and brain active with sounds, and relying on a hearing aid is a positive step.

Since your hearing loss happened gradually, you might not have noticed big changes from day to day. However, after getting used to hearing well with a hearing aid, you'll likely notice a bigger difference (not hearing as well) when you take it off.

7# MYTH:

My hearing loss isn't severe enough for a hearing aid.

FACT: When you have hearing loss in some frequencies and not others, it is easier to dismiss it as unimportant. However, even mild hearing loss can adversely affect your cognitive capabilities, work, home, and social life.

FACTS

Some unique facts and data shed light on the challenges and opportunities faced by the deaf community in India and around the world:

1# Deafness means having trouble hearing. Around 466 million people worldwide experience some level of hearing difficulty.

2# Only about 10% of deaf children in India have access to education, and even fewer receive proper language and communication support.

3# Gallaudet University in the United States is the only university in the world designed specifically to cater to the educational needs of deaf and hard-of-hearing students.

4# Indian Sign Language (ISL) is not widely recognized or taught in educational institutions, limiting communication and educational opportunities for deaf individuals.

5# The Rights of Persons with Disabilities Act (RPwD), passed in 2016, includes provisions for the rights of deaf individuals and mandates the promotion of Indian Sign Language.

6# Deaf people can feel music and sounds through vibrations. If you put your hand on a speaker, you can feel the thumping beats of music–that's how deaf people often "hear".

7# Imran Sheikh known as the (Dhoni Of the India Deaf Cricket Team) has represented India in the Deaf Cricket World Cup. He has shown that determination and skill can lead to success in the world of sports.

SUMMARY

The book "Silent Epidemic" talks about hearing and its importance. It starts by telling us about a special hospital called Satkriti Hospitals Private Limited. This hospital's name means doing good things for people. It was founded by doctors who know a lot about ears, nose, and throat problems, as well as diabetes. This hospital is located in the middle of the city of Varanasi (one of the world's oldest continually inhabited cities) and helps people who have problems with their ears, nose, throat, deafness, and diabetes.

The book then tells us about deafness, which is when someone can't hear properly. It can happen because of different reasons like family history, getting older, loud noises, infection and diseases. The book explains how important it is to protect our ears and not listen to sounds that can hurt them. This book also enlightens readers about the importance of safe hearing practices.

The book also talks about ways to communicate if someone can't hear well, suggesting the use of devices to help hear better. It's important to know about deafness so we can prevent it and help people who have it. The book gives tips to keep our ears safe, like paying attention if our ears feel strange and talking to a doctor if they ring a lot. It also talks about yoga, which can help keep our ears healthy.

The book has different chapters that cover topics like how loud noises can be harmful, the social side of not hearing well, and what to do if someone suddenly can't hear.

My Vision

Freedom From Deafness

Deaf Free India by 2047

I envision a world free from deafness, and I am dedicated to making this vision a reality in India by 2047. Collaborating with a network of doctors, researchers, and communities across the country, our mission is multifaceted. We are committed to raising awareness about hearing health, implementing early intervention programs, and advancing medical treatments. Our goal is to ensure accessible and quality healthcare for everyone, leveraging new technologies to facilitate broader inclusion.

Through strategic partnerships with organizations that share our vision, we aim to set measurable targets for the reduction of hearing problems, focusing on specific age groups and regions. We recognize the transformative power of technology and are actively incorporating innovative solutions to enhance healthcare and communication for individuals with hearing difficulties.

Our mission is rooted in the principle of inclusion. We believe that everyone, regardless of their hearing abilities, should have equal opportunities to participate in all aspects of life. While the journey ahead is challenging, we are confident that our collective efforts will lead to a future where hearing problems are significantly reduced, and everyone can enjoy the gift of hearing and seamless communication.

CONNECT WITH US

Dear Reader,

As we reach the end of this book, I would like to express my deepest gratitude for taking the time to read it.

I would be thrilled to hear about your experiences and the transformations you undergo after implementing the principles shared within these pages. Your feedback is invaluable and will greatly contribute to my ongoing work and future publications.

Also, as part of my service mission to create a Deafness-Free Nation, I am committed to doing whatever I can. And, you, dear reader, can be my ambassadors in this mission. While my reach is limited on my own, with you as my eyes and ears, we can truly make a difference.

If you come across or know of any child who is less than 5 years old and is unable to speak or hear, please refer that child to our hospital, irrespective of their economic background.

If the child is under 5 years old, does not have any associated abnormalities, and the parents are financially weak and unable to afford the cost of the surgery, we can provide the surgery free of cost, along with 1 year of post-surgery speech therapy and rehabilitation. (Normally, the surgery costs around 8-10 lakhs for each ear).

Let deafness not be a barrier to living a full and happy life. Schedule a diagnostic appointment with our team for any hearing-related issues or guidance of hearing aids. Together, we can help everyone hear & dance to the divine music of life.

You can connect with me at: ***manoj2061@gmail.com***

website: ***satkritihospital.com***

WhatsApp No.: ***9455959800***

For Appointment: ***Call us at 8765848001***

Drop a Mail: ***care.satkriti@gmail.com***

Let's go on this journey together to make a world where everyone can hear and live better by connecting with each other through the sounds of love.

Warm regards,

Dr. Manoj Kumar Gupta

MBBS, M.S(ENT) Chief ENT Consultant & Founder Director

(Formerly At AIIMS, New Delhi)

Satkriti Hospitals Private Limited

Varanasi - 221005,India

Youtube Channel Link

Google Map Scanner

Facebook

www.ingramcontent.com/pod-product-compliance
Ingram Content Group UK Ltd.
Pitfield, Milton Keynes, MK11 3LW, UK
UKHW021656190726
13853UKWH00001B/288

9 789355 549518